I0464975

CAREER AS A

RADIATION THERAPIST

RADIATION IS ONE OF THE MOST powerful forces known to man. In comics and the movies, radiation transforms ordinary people into super heroes. In the real world, radiation can be very dangerous. Nations threaten each other with nuclear bombs and the consequences of a meltdown at a nuclear power plant can be catastrophic. But the power of radiation can also be a lifesaver. When targeted at a tumor, it can give cancer victims back their lives.

Radiation therapy is critical in the fight against cancer. More than one million Americans are diagnosed with cancer each year. It is estimated that about half of them receive radiation therapy as part of their treatment. Radiation may be used alone or in conjunction with surgery, chemotherapy or other forms of cancer therapy.

Radiation therapy is also known as radiotherapy, x-ray therapy, electron beam therapy, cobalt therapy, or irradiation. Whatever term you use, it is a treatment that uses high-energy x-rays, targeted at a tumor, to help shrink or eliminate cancerous tissue. Sometimes tumors are considered inoperable because of their size. Radiation therapy can be used to shrink them down to a manageable size so that they can be surgically removed. The treatment is also commonly used following surgery to destroy any cancer cells that were not removed by surgery. When a cure is not possible, radiation can be used to help relieve the symptoms of advanced cancer (such as bleeding or pain).

The radiation for cancer treatment comes from special machines operated by radiation therapists. These professionals work as members of an entire oncology (cancer) team, performing many other important duties during the planning and treatment process. For example, they use an x-ray machine or computer tomography (CT) scan to pinpoint the tumor, monitor patients' physical and emotional well-being during treatment, and keep meticulous records that may be used for research purposes.

In addition to medical knowledge of the radiation process, radiation therapists must possess excellent communications skills. It can be difficult to be empathetic and compassionate toward patients without becoming overwhelmed with emotion. Radiation therapy can save a cancer patient's life, but in some cases the treatment is ineffective, or even makes the cancer worse. Some radiation therapists find their job emotionally grueling because of the high stakes, but most find it incredibly rewarding.

Most (about 70 percent) radiation therapists work in hospitals or in cancer treatment centers. Others work in physicians' offices as assistants, and a small number work in outpatient care centers and medical and diagnostic laboratories performing research. Across all practice settings, job opportunities for radiation therapists are expected to increase dramatically. As the population in the United States ages and develops higher risks for cancer, the demand grows. As radiation technology becomes safer and more effective, it will be prescribed more often, leading to even more jobs for radiation therapists.

Considering the attractive features of this career – good pay and great job outlook – the educational requirements are quite modest. There are two ways to get the necessary training. One is by obtaining an associate or a bachelor's degree in radiation therapy. The other is to go through a certificate program, which generally takes less time than the full four years of an undergraduate degree. Prospective radiation therapists should make sure that their degree or certificate program is certified by the American Registry of Radiologic Technologists (ARRT) before they enroll.

Once radiation therapists begin working, their earnings are fairly high. Beginners start out with salaries of $50,000 per year on average. Their earnings rise the longer they stay in the job – those with 10 year's experience typically make $75,000 to $85,000 per year. Some make even more working at specialty hospitals or in medical and diagnostic laboratories.

The greatest reward of working as a radiation therapist is witnessing the scientific advances that allow many cancer patients to survive and go back to leading healthy lives. It was just over 100 years ago that the German physicist Wilhelm Roentgen discovered x-rays and the scientist Marie Curie discovered the radioactive element radium. Their discoveries began a new era in medical treatment and research. Radiation therapy techniques have improved dramatically, especially in recent years. Radiation therapists get to watch from the front lines as treatment techniques continue to advance. They have the satisfaction of knowing that their work makes a profound difference in patients' lives.

If you are detail oriented, good at communication, and enjoy being physically, emotionally, and intellectually challenged, radiation therapy may be a good career choice for you.

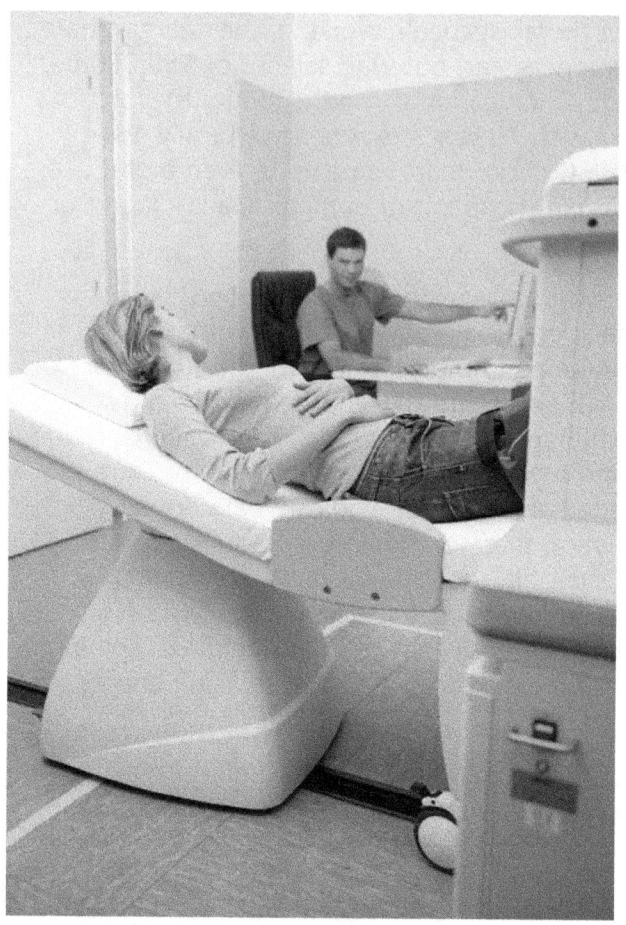

YOUR ASSIGNMENT

A CAREER IN RADIATION THERAPY requires intensive education. You should talk to your guidance counselor to get help putting together a curriculum that satisfies college entrance requirements. Research different colleges, look over their catalogs, and make sure you are doing everything necessary to prepare.

This is a highly technical career involving math and science. Take courses in physics, pre-calculus, algebra, computer science, research methodology, human anatomy, and physiology. The more you load up on these type of courses, the better your chances of being accepted into a radiation therapy program.

Radiation therapists also need good communications skills because they interact on a daily basis with cancer patients. Check to see what kind of communications classes your high school offers. Writing, public speaking, debate, or even drama classes can be helpful. Even better, consider volunteering at a hospital where you can watch radiation therapists in action and get accustomed to being around patients.

To get a good idea of what this type of work is all about, talk to the professionals. Contact radiation therapists directly to ask about their typical work day. Ask what they like and dislike about their job. Ask why they chose this career and what school they went to. Different therapists will have different experiences and opinions, so get information from as many as you can.

Start researching radiation therapy on the Internet. RTstudents.com is a radiation therapy website that lists helpful links for schools and jobs. The Mayo Clinic and the American Registry of Radiologic Technologists can also answer many of your questions about the profession.

HISTORY OF THE CAREER

THE FIELD OF RADIATION THERAPY was born in 1895 when German physicist, Wilhelm Roentgen, made an exciting new discovery. While conducting electrical experiments, Roentgen noticed an energy ray that could pass through his own body. He soon realized that these rays, which he named "x-rays," could be used to produce images of bones – something no one had imagined before.

The next big step in the field occurred a few years later. In

1898, scientist Marie Curie discovered the radioactive element radium. Together, Roentgen's and Curie's discoveries created a stir in the scientific community, and a new era in medical treatment and research took off. Scientists quickly learned that radium and x-rays caused hair loss and skin damage. They also observed that these same destructive forces could treat superficial skin diseases and unwanted hair. It was only by chance that doctors discovered radiation could regress or slow down the growth of some tumors. They did not understand why radiation worked in that way, but the first radiation therapists went on to cure their first cancer case in 1898.

The cancers treated by radiation in the early 1900s were superficial and a high rate of recurring tumors was common. The problem was the imprecision of treatment techniques and the lack of medical knowledge concerning radiation and cancer. It had only been a few short years since the discovery of radiation after all. Researchers were hard at work unlocking the mysteries of this new therapy and great improvements were close at hand.

By 1913, doctors advanced from treating skin cancer to other superficial cancers like head, breast, and neck lymph nodes. Radium was being mined in America, and General Electric created a 140 KV (kilovolt) tube for storing it. Doctors were now able to insert small tubes of the rare and expensive radium directly into cancers or into body cavities containing cancer. Radium made it possible, for example, to cure inoperable cervical cancer for the first time.

In 1922, General Electric developed special x-ray tubes with high energy (200 KV) for deeply imbedded lung, abdominal, and pelvic tumors. After that, inoperable larynx cancer became curable. In the United States, surgery remained the preferred cancer therapy with radiation reserved for inoperable or recurrent tumors. Radiation therapy came to be known as the "last hope" in the process of cancer treatment.

Between World Wars I and II, scientists continued to study how radiation works and how to measure the dose more accurately. Physicists, electrical engineers, mining companies, and commercial vendors developed and marketed higher energy x-ray machines and new radium devices. After World War II, particle accelerators and nuclear reactors became available to produce synthetic radium and other radioactive elements for cancer treatment. The first cobalt machine, using synthetic radium, appeared in 1951. Within the first 10 years of its invention, 1,120 cobalt machines were sold to hospitals around the world.

Radiation research and hardware advances led to the creation of the medical linear accelerator x-ray machine in 1953. This is the same technology that is still used today in the treatment of cancer. Charged particles are propelled through a vacuum tunnel called a linac, or linear accelerator. This allows the x-rays to penetrate concentrated cancerous areas deep in the body while not affecting the healthy skin tissue as much.

Scientists Henry Kaplan and Edward Ginzton from Stanford University worked together to improve the linear accelerator to a standard where it could be used in a clinical setting. By 1960, they had created the first publicly launched rotational radiation therapy linear accelerator. They named it a linac.

The linear accelerator quickly progressed from 4 MV energy to 18 MV and began to dominate the market. Both the cobalt machines and the high-energy linacs improved cancer cure rates dramatically. Previously incurable Hodgkin's lymphomas and testicle cancers became curable. However, the linear accelerator's accuracy in locating tumors and directing charged particles was still inexact.

The biggest goal in developing better radiation therapy hardware was to prevent the radiation from affecting healthy cells as much as possible. The tumor had to be targeted more accurately and the charged particles needed to match the tumor's shape. In 1971, Godfrey Hounsfield invented computed tomography (CT), which facilitated the shift from 2-D to 3-D radiation delivery. CT-based planning allowed doctors to measure the radiation dose based on axial tomographical images – three-dimensional images that defined normal and abnormal objects in the body. Godfrey Hounsfield's discovery is still used by doctors today in three-dimensional conformal radiation therapy (3DCRT).

The more advanced form of 3DCRT is intensity-modulated radiation therapy (IMRT). In the late 1980s, only a handful of physicists worldwide were studying how to use IMRT to map information from CT scans to produce 3-D images of tumors. But IMRT developed so rapidly that its recent past is also its ancient history.

IMRT planning is conceptually distinct from conventional radiation therapy planning. With IMRT, image data is fed into the x-ray beam linear accelerator system to target the contours of the tumor. Beams are then automatically adjusted to hit only cancerous tissue in highly controlled doses. The goal is to reduce the amount of radiation hitting healthy tissues while delivering a full dose of radiation to the tumors. The healthy tissues remain functional and mostly undamaged; the tumors are destroyed.

A recent specific form of IMRT is the TomoTherapy system. TomoTherapy system is a commercial, patented process that uses the CT guided IMRT technology to direct the radiation source spiraling around the patient. This makes the 3-D contours of a tumor more easily traced by the beam from the linear accelerator. TomoTherapy had its first clinical use in 2003.

The latest advancement in scanning technology for radiation therapy is a system called Image Guided Radiation Treatment (IGRT). One of the most significant setbacks in scanning and targeting tumors had been the movements tumors make when the patient breathes or shifts during treatment. The

IGRT machine compensates for any movement the tumor may have by using high resolution x-rays to produce images that highlight the contrast between cancerous tumors and the healthy surrounding tissue. These images allow doctors to target the tumor more precisely, ensuring that only the less healthy tissues are exposed to radiation.

The progression of radiation therapy over time has improved the efficacy and accessibility of cancer treatment. Of course, cancer remains a pressing medical issue. Scientists and doctors continue to push beyond what they have already achieved. New breakthroughs in the study and field of radiation therapy will be essential in the fight to cure cancer.

WHERE YOU WILL WORK

ABOUT 70 PERCENT OF RADIATION therapists work in hospitals or in cancer treatment centers. Cancer treatment facilities exist all over the world, but most are found in regions that are developed enough to have the necessary high tech equipment and highly trained staff.

About 20 percent of radiation therapists work as assistants in physicians' offices and outpatient care centers. A small number are employed by medical and diagnostic laboratories to perform research. Some very experienced radiation therapists leave their clinical surroundings for academia, to teach in medical schools or radiation therapy certification programs.

In some countries, radiation therapists can also work as medical dosimetrists. (Dosimetrists calculate the amount of radium needed in a dose using complex mathematical formulas.) In the United States, however, radiation therapists must obtain certification in dosimetry in addition to their radiation therapy certification before they can work as dosimetrists.

Radiation therapists working in cancer treatment centers and hospitals generally work in teams. The radiation oncology team usually includes a primary care physician, a radiation oncologist, a dosimetrist, a radiation therapist, an oncology nurse, and a medical physicist.

There are few opportunities for travel in this profession. Because cancer treatment requires many different specialists working in collaboration, radiation therapists can't travel alone to provide medical volunteer work in other countries.

The hospitals, cancer treatment centers, outpatient centers, and medical laboratories that radiation therapists work in are generally clean, well lit, and well ventilated. They are equipped with high tech machines and very advanced computer hardware and software.

Because they work around radioactive materials, radiation therapists take great care to ensure that they are not exposed to dangerous levels of radiation. By following standard safety procedures, radiation therapists can prevent overexposure. Even pregnant women are allowed to work as radiation therapists.

The work can be fairly physical, because you are constantly lifting and positioning disabled patients on and off of treatment tables. Therapists also move back and forth between the treatment room and the radiation-secure room where they operate equipment and monitor patients. Radiation therapists spend most of the work day on their feet.

Work schedules for radiation therapists are ordinary and stable. Overtime and night shifts are rare. The workweek is the typical 40 hours. Unlike employees in many other health-care occupations, radiation therapists usually work only during the day. Nonetheless, radiation therapy emergencies do occur. Some therapists are required to be on call and may have to work outside of their normal hours.

THE WORK YOU WILL DO

RADIATION THERAPISTS USE machines called linear accelerators to administer radiation treatment to cancer patients. They work alongside several members of a medical radiation oncology team (oncology means the study of tumors). Radiation therapists' duties include the following:

Operate an x-ray imaging machine or computer tomography (CT) scan

Perform simulations before delivering actual treatments

Position patients so that treatments can be delivered accurately

Help dosimetrists calculate the optimal radiation dosage

Monitor patients' physical and emotional well-being during treatment

Communicate with patients before and during treatment

Explain treatment plans to patients and their families

Operate the linear accelerator

The Radiation Oncology Team

Radiation therapy is not a treatment that can be handled by one person – no matter how highly trained that individual might be. It takes an entire team of specialists. In addition to the radiation therapist, this team usually includes the following medical professionals:

Radiation oncologist – is the doctor who specializes in using radiation to treat cancer. Generally considered the team leader, the radiation oncologist is responsible for prescribing the type and amount of treatment for each patient.

Radiation physicist – is in charge of the main piece of

equipment used in radiation therapy, the linear accelerator. This individual works closely with the radiation oncologist to plan the patient's treatment, then makes sure the machine is delivering the correct amount of radiation. The physicist's responsibilities include making sure the linear accelerator is working properly, making adjustments when calibrations are off, and checking the machine for safety.

Dosimetrist – works under the direction of the radiation oncologist and the physicist. The dosimetrist's primary responsibility is to calculate the amount of radiation that will be targeting the cancer and how much will be delivered to surrounding normal tissues.

Radiation oncology nurses – are registered nurses (RNs) who are specifically trained to deal with oncology patients. They coordinate patient care and (along with radiation therapists) educate patients and their families so they understand what to expect. Radiation oncology nurses have a tough job – they are the ones who are responsible for managing patients' side effects from the radiation treatments.

Support staff – include various individuals who sign in patients upon arrival and make the daily operations run smoothly.

The Process

Before beginning treatment, the radiation oncology team must come up with a treatment plan. To create this plan, the radiation therapist must first use three-dimensional imaging to pinpoint the exact location of the tumor (or abnormality) and define its exact size and shape. Computer tomography (CT), MRI, and PET/CT can be used for these scans, but CT is the most common.

The CT scans allow the radiation oncology team to view images of the tumor in 3-D. The radiation oncologist and the radiation physicist use the images from the scans to determine the best way to administer treatment. The treatment plan is specific and detailed. It spells out which beams of radiation will converge on the target area from different angles and planes as well as the careful positioning of the patient for therapy sessions.

The radiation therapist then positions the patient and adjusts the linear accelerator as directed by the specifications in the treatment plan. During this time, the radiation therapist must also record details so that these conditions can be exactly replicated during treatment. The radiation therapist explains the treatment plan to the patient and answers any questions the patient might have.

If a patient opts for a full simulation of treatment, the radiation therapist places the patient in the treatment position on a special x-ray machine or computer tomography scanner and takes simulation x-rays. Masks, pads, or other devices may be used to help the patient hold still in one position during the simulation.

After completing the treatment plan and simulation, the actual treatment begins. Treatment can take anywhere from 10 to 30 minutes. The radiation therapist follows the detailed guidelines developed during the planning process to position the patient. Then, the therapist adjusts and operates the linear accelerator.

The linear accelerator stays in a room with lead and concrete walls so that the high-energy x-rays are shielded. The radiation therapist must turn on the accelerator from outside the treatment room. Because the accelerator only gives off radiation when it is actually turned on, the risk of accidental exposure is extremely low.

During treatment the radiation therapist continuously watches the patient through a closed-circuit television monitor. There is also a microphone in the treatment room so that the patient can speak to the therapist if needed. Port films (x-rays taken with the treatment beam) and other imaging tools are checked regularly to make sure that the beam position doesn't vary from the original plan developed by the oncology team.

Throughout the treatment, the radiation therapist monitors the patient's physical condition to determine whether the patient is having any adverse reactions. The radiation therapist must also be aware of the patient's emotional well-being. Because many patients feel stressed by the treatment, the radiation therapist must provide emotional support as well.

The radiation therapist positions and controls linear accelerators in a procedure called external beam therapy. Linear accelerators use powerful generators to project high energy x-rays at targeted cancer cells. The linear accelerator can be used to treat all parts and organs of the body. It has a special set of lead shutters, called collimators, which focus and direct a uniform dose of high-energy x-ray to the region of the patient's tumor. As the x-rays intersect with human tissue, they produce highly energized ions that damage the DNA of cancerous cells. These x-rays destroy the cancer cells while sparing the surrounding normal tissue.

Linear accelerators are also used for Intensity-Modulated Radiation Therapy (IMRT), Image-Guided Radiation Therapy (IGRT), and Stereotactic Radiosurgery (SRS). Radiation therapists are involved in these treatments as well. Before beginning an IMRT, IGRT, or SRS treatment, the radiation therapist positions the patient on the treatment table, and then, as with external beam therapy, the radiation therapist operates the equipment from a radiation-protected area nearby.

IMRT is a precise and highly advanced mode of radiation therapy. The IMRT uses mapping information from CT scans to produce a 3-D image of the tumor. The image data is then fed into the x-ray beam linear accelerator system to target the contours of the tumor. IMRT allows for the radiation dose to conform more precisely to the three-dimensional shape of the tumor by modulating the intensity of the radiation beam in multiple small volumes. IMRT also allows higher radiation doses to be focused on regions within the tumor while minimizing the dose to surrounding normal critical structures, making it a highly efficient treatment.

IGRT is the use of frequent imaging during a course of radiation therapy to improve the precision and accuracy of the treatment. IGRT is used to treat tumors in areas of the body that are prone to movement, such as the lungs (which move when the patient breathes) and prostate gland, as well as tumors located close to critical organs and tissues.

SRS is another highly efficient form of radiation therapy. Despite its name, stereotactic radiosurgery is a non-surgical procedure that delivers precisely-targeted radiation at much higher doses than traditional radiation therapy while sparing healthy tissue organs nearby. Stereotactic radiosurgery relies on several technologies.

Safety

One of the most important responsibilities assigned to radiation therapists is ensuring patient safety. After all, radiation is dangerous and can even be deadly if misused. Radiation therapists check the radiation machines and linear accelerators for safety and accuracy before each treatment to make sure they are working properly. If there is any anomaly, they call upon the radiation physicist for assistance.

To ensure additional safety, there are several systems built into the linear accelerator and radiation machines so that it won't deliver a higher dose than the radiation oncologist prescribed. Modern radiation machines have internal checking systems to provide further safety so that the machine will not turn on until all the treatment requirements prescribed by the oncology team have been accurately completed. When all the checks match and are accurate, the radiation therapist can turn the machine on to administer treatment.

During treatment, therapists monitor the patient as well as the machine. They use a piece of equipment called a "tracker" to ensure that the radiation intensity is uniform across the beam.

Keeping Records

Before, during, and after treatment, radiation therapists must keep detailed records. These records include the following information:

Patient positioning details

Dose of radiation used for each treatment

Total amount of radiation used to date

The area treated

The patient's reactions

The radiation therapist's records must be accurate because radiation oncologists and dosimetrists review the records to evaluate whether the treatment plan is working. The records are also used to monitor the amount of radiation exposure that the patient has received, and to minimize side effects.

Advancement

An experienced radiation therapist may be asked to assist the dosimetrist. After the physician consults with the patient on their plan of treatment, the radiation oncologist writes a prescription dose to a defined tumor volume. The dosimetrist then designs a treatment plan using a computer or manual computation that will deliver that prescribed radiation dose. The radiation therapist may then help the dosimetrist in calculating that dosage.

With additional training and certification, radiation therapists can advance to become dosimetrists themselves. Other advancement opportunities for radiation therapists include teaching, technical sales, or research. Experienced radiation therapists may also advance to manage radiation therapy programs in treatment centers or other healthcare facilities. Manager radiation therapists generally continue to treat patients while taking on management responsibilities.

STORIES OF PEOPLE IN THE CAREER

I Work in a Cancer Research Center

"I always knew that my career would have something to do with medicine because both my parents were in the medical world. My father was a doctor, but ultimately it was my mother who influenced me the most. She was deeply involved in cancer research.

Unlike many other research positions, my work involves constant interaction with people. I work as part of a team of radiation therapists treating cancer patients. I also work closely with specific physicians to help develop and implement their research protocols. I also have the opportunity to maintain close contact with a number of patients and their families. It was during an internship that I was able to develop the high level of personal skills necessary to interact effectively with all these different people.

Of course, highly specialized technical skills are also needed for this kind of work. My training included an intensive curriculum that prepared me to implement treatment programs prescribed by a radiation oncologist. As you can imagine, there is a considerable amount of technology involved. For example, I use the computer tomography (CT) scanner to plan the treatments and then operate the linear accelerator to deliver the radiation during treatments.

My typical workday is extremely busy because a new patient comes in every 15 minutes. I am responsible for scheduling and treating my own patients. Each patient is treated Monday to Friday for about six weeks. In addition to the actual treatment, there is a lot of paperwork to be done – therapy charts, daily records of treatment, and quality assurance reviews.

The best thing about my job is being able to work directly with the patients. I don't think I would like being isolated in a lab peering into a microscope all day. I need to know that what I am doing is making a difference in the lives of real people. A big part of my job is to educate the patients and their families, and provide support. In this position, I am able to make an unpleasant and complicated situation much easier for them. On my best days, I turn fear into hope. That is the most rewarding aspect of my career.

The only thing I don't like about my work is that it is necessary at all. I truly hope we find a cure for all cancers and that my profession will no longer be needed. Until that day comes, research as a radiation therapist will continue to be filled with challenges and opportunities. I am very proud of my contributions, however small. I know my input is valued and important."

I Teach Radiation Therapy at a University Hospital

"Like many people who have chosen to pursue healthcare careers, my motivation came from personal experience. My mother died of ovarian cancer when I was 20. She was diagnosed with cancer when I was a senior in high school. I went with her to many of her cancer treatments and became quite familiar with the different people who worked with her and other cancer patients. Although I started out my college education as an English lit major, I changed course after my mother's death. Cancer changes the lives of people it touches in profound ways. For me, the battle against this dreadful disease became my life's work. I chose a career in radiation therapy.

Radiation therapy is intense work that requires an equal level of cognitive skills and emotional intelligence. A radiation therapist has to be at the top of the game every minute of the day. The day moves fast. Typically, a new patient is treated every 15 minutes. That's four patients per hour, upwards of 30 per day. The radiation therapist can't rush through each treatment session. You must carefully deliver treatment, evaluate the patient's response, assess a number of parameters, and keep meticulous records of it all.

Because a patient can only receive a limited amount of radiation dose each day, it can take anywhere from two to eight weeks for a patient to complete the treatment regimen. During that time the radiation therapist works with the patient and the family every day. You must be part educator, part cheerleader. This is naturally an intensely emotional time for everyone involved. It takes a special kind of person to handle it calmly without seeming cold and detached. The challenge is to offer steady reassurance without giving false hope.

After 10 years working as a radiation therapist, I decided to become a teacher. I saw that the need for trained therapists is growing rapidly and felt I could help more patients by helping students get that training. I already had an undergraduate degree in radiologic science with certifications in radiation therapy, medical imaging, and dosimetry. I went back to school to earn a master's degree in healthcare administration and a doctorate in higher education administration.

Today, my favorite activity is giving talks at high schools. I don't limit my discussions to the nuts and bolts of radiation therapy and how it works. What will inspire young people to enter the profession is the realization that this work benefits people. It is a thrill to run into patients I treated years ago and see how happy and healthy they are today.

My advice to young people thinking of getting into radiation therapy is first to discuss it with their guidance counselor. The counselor can help them prepare for their college education. They should also talk to professionals in the field. There are local chapters of the American Society of Radiologic Technologists all over the country. Contacting them is the best way to learn about the profession.

My work as a radiation therapy teacher has been incredibly rewarding. I am so proud of every graduate who has gone on to help cure cancer. They have touched many lives with their noble work."

PERSONAL QUALIFICATIONS

TO BE SUCCESSFUL AS A RADIATION therapist you must possess many personal qualifications beyond what is taught in the classroom. Are you detail oriented, a team player with a head for math and scientific aptitude? Are you both emotionally and physically fit – empathetic and psychologically capable of working with people who have cancer, while coordinated enough to handle machinery and disabled patients? If so, you possess the basic requirements.

Radiation therapists need special communications and interactive skills. In fact, people applying for jobs as radiation therapists are evaluated more and more on the basis of their communications skills and emotional intelligence than on their technical expertise. Learning to operate the equipment is the easy part. The hard part is interacting on a daily basis with patients who are sick and stressed and who know they may not get better. It requires enormous patience and compassion towards patients, while not being overwhelmed with emotion. It is a balancing act that can create stress, and not everyone can handle it.

Radiation treatment is painless, but it can cause a number of side effects in patients including fatigue, nausea, hair loss, and skin reactions. In rare cases, radiation can also cause cancer. Some patients experience secondary malignancies as a result of radiation therapy. For these reasons, radiation therapy can be stressful, even traumatic, for patients and their loved ones. Being around those sorts of situations on a regular basis can be emotionally grueling for radiation therapists.

In addition to being emotionally stable, you must also be

physically fit. It takes strength and coordination to accurately position medical equipment while lifting and situating disabled patients. You must also be able to spend much of your work day on your feet. Because radiation therapists help evaluate 3D images of tumors, good eyesight and normal color vision are necessary.

Are you good at keeping accurate, detailed records? There is a surprising amount of paperwork involved in this work. Radiation therapists record patient and treatment information every day that is vital for ensuring patient safety and treatment effectiveness. They take notes concerning the patient's position on the treatment table, the tumor measurements, the radiation dosage, the medical equipment settings, the treatment length, and the patient's reactions to treatment. They record this information as they are moving around, operating equipment, and interacting with patients – a juggling act that requires multitasking skills.

You must be able to work equally well one-on-one and in groups. Radiation therapists interact directly with patients all day. Many of the duties are done with little or no supervision. You must have the skills and confidence necessary to work without someone looking over your shoulder. You should be comfortable operating equipment and dealing with patients on your own.

This is not a solitary profession. Radiation therapists are part of a team of radiation oncology professionals. You must understand the doctor-patient relationship and how to behave as a member of a medical team. Most of your team members will be in a higher position of authority than you, so you must respect that authority and be comfortable with following orders. However, this does not mean your voice will not be heard. After all, you are also a highly trained professional. You should have the confidence to express your opinions to your superiors when you feel it is necessary.

ATTRACTIVE FEATURES

RADIATION THERAPY IS A PROFESSION with many attractive features. To begin with, the job outlook is much better for radiation therapy than for most other professions. As the population in the United States ages, jobs for radiation therapists grow. Radiation therapy careers are projected to increase by a whopping 27 percent over the next decade.

You can also make good money in this career. Entry-level radiation therapists who have worked in the field for one year or less have a median salary of about $50,000 per year. That is an excellent starting salary and earnings increase the longer you stay at the job. Radiation therapists with five to nine years of job experience have salaries of about $65,000 per year, and those with 10 years or more experience typically can make up to $85,000 per year. There is also room for upward mobility, either by moving into teaching or research positions, or working as a medical dosimetrist.

The amount of education and training required to be a radiation therapist is not as great as for other healthcare professions. You do not have to attend medical school. You are only required to complete an associate or a bachelor's degree program in radiation therapy and pass a certification examination.

Although there is little opportunity for travel, radiation therapists do have a certain amount of job mobility. They can work in hospitals, outpatient care centers, physicians' offices, universities, and medical laboratories just about anywhere in the country.

No matter where you work as a radiation therapist, you can expect good working conditions. Hospitals, clinics, and cancer treatment centers are clean, well lit, well ventilated, and equipped with top-of-the-line computers and radiation equipment. Unlike other healthcare workers, radiation therapists almost never have to work at night or put in overtime. You can expect a regular 35 to 40 hour workweek.

As a radiation therapist you can expect a great benefits package in addition to your salary. You will almost certainly receive healthcare coverage, paid holidays, vacation time, and a retirement plan. You may even receive life insurance or disability and paid sick leave, reimbursement for education or training costs, and malpractice insurance.

Radiation therapists get to be physically active during the work day. Instead of sitting at a desk, you will be on the go, moving around to position patients and equipment. This may help you feel healthier and more energetic at the end of your shift.

One of the best parts about being a radiation therapist is that you have the opportunity to make a positive difference in the lives of cancer patients and their loved ones. Your patients are depending on you to make them healthy again, and they are so grateful when you do. You will always have the satisfaction of knowing that on a daily basis you make a profound difference in people's lives.

As a radiation therapist you also get to be around smart and motivated people who have interests and goals similar to yours. When facing a challenging treatment plan, you will know that you have the support of your team. Because you work closely together every day, you will likely form lasting friendships with some of your co-workers.

UNATTRACTIVE FEATURES

SOME OF THE BEST THINGS ABOUT working as a radiation therapist can also be the worst. Interacting with cancer patients each and every day can leave some radiation therapists feeling depressed. Because radiation therapy is a high risk procedure (sometimes it can increase the number of times tumors recur or actually cause cancer), radiation therapists are under great pressure to do their job perfectly. It is a sad reality that there is no way to guarantee a successful outcome. No matter how well radiation therapists perform all their duties, some cancer patients will get worse. All radiation therapists have to face the possibility that patients who come in for treatment expecting to be cured may in fact end up worse off than before they came in.

Radiation therapists are constantly interacting with patients and consulting with the rest of the radiation oncology team. This lack of autonomy can be tiresome for those who would rather work alone. Radiation therapists have less authority than other members of the radiation oncology team. They must follow the instructions given by their superiors, which can be frustrating for those who are natural leaders and like to be in charge. If radiation therapists don't like their co-workers on a personal level, they most likely won't be able to switch to a different radiation oncology team unless they are based in a big treatment center.

This is surprisingly physical work. Daily activities can be quite strenuous. Radiation therapists are constantly lifting and positioning disabled patients, positioning medical equipment, and walking to and from the treatment room to the monitoring room. This can be difficult for anyone with a disability that hinders movement.

Some healthcare workers enjoy a rotational schedule that concentrates work into longer, but fewer shifts, allowing longer chunks of time off. Radiation therapists work a regular, 40 hour a week job which some may find monotonous and inflexible. Also, the work tends to be routine, with a limited number of tasks to perform over and over.

Job mobility for radiation therapists is limited by the fact that licensure is different from state to state. This means that radiation therapists may have to pass a new state licensure exam for every state they move to.

The education required to be a radiation therapist involves math, science, and computer skills. This can be difficult for those who don't excel in those subjects. You might have the right emotional intelligence for the job, but without the technical aptitude, the prerequisite training will seem tough.

Unlike healthcare workers who are able to provide medical volunteer work abroad with minimal facilities and assistance, radiation therapists are bound to their facilities. They are always dependent upon the rest of the radiation oncology team and upon state-of-the-art equipment to be able to do their work.

EDUCATION AND TRAINING

ASPIRING RADIATION THERAPISTS are usually required to complete an associate or a bachelor's degree program in radiation therapy. However, they may also become qualified by completing an associate or a bachelor's degree program in radiography (the study of radiological imaging), followed by a year-long certificate program in radiation therapy.

Students with little or no experience in the radiation therapy field typically enter a traditional degree program. These programs usually require freshman and sophomores to complete a general education curriculum before specializing in radiation therapy in their junior year.

There are also certificate programs in radiation therapy that require less time than the full four years of an undergraduate degree. These programs tend to be narrowly focused, concentrating only on the subjects students should know for certification and licensure. This is an option generally reserved for candidates with experience in medical imaging or similar work.

Most accredited radiation therapy programs offer courses in anatomy and physiology, social sciences and humanities, introduction to radiation therapy and oncology, caring for a patient at the end of life, radiobiology, human relations, radiology technology and therapy techniques. The diversity of courses gives students a strong educational foundation and allows them to determine if they want to specialize in a given area.

Lab instruction is also an important factor in radiation therapy programs. Most schools require a set number of hours of clinical experience through volunteer hours in cancer centers, cooperating hospitals, and medical centers.

Selecting a program that is accredited by the American Registry of Radiologic Technologists (ARRT) is important. Studying in an accredited program is a requirement for certification in radiation therapy. The Joint Review Committee on Education in Radiologic Technology (JRCERT), an agency for radiation therapists that is recognized by the United States Department of Education, lists the accredited programs for radiation therapy. There are about 100 accredited radiation therapy programs in the US. With so many accredited programs across the country, candidates for radiation therapy have a good chance of finding the type of program that most interests them in the state where they wish to live and work.

Admissions to both certificate and bachelor's degree radiation therapy programs are limited and selective, and some require visits to hospitals before consideration. After completion, a certification exam must be passed to enter the field.

Certification

Some states, as well as many employers, require radiation therapists to be certified by The American Association of Radiologic Technologists (ARRT). To become ARRT-certified, the applicant must complete an accredited radiation therapy program, agree to adhere to ARRT ethical standards, and pass the ARRT certification examination.

The certification examination is a computer-based test that is offered several times throughout the year at various locations. The certification examination tests a candidate's knowledge of radiation protection and quality assurance, clinical concepts in radiation oncology, treatment planning, treatment delivery, and patient care and education. Candidates must also demonstrate competency in several clinical practices including patient care activities, simulation procedures, dosimetry calculations, and the application of radiation. Once the test is passed, those who graduate from an accredited program can call themselves registered radiation therapists.

ARRT certification is valid for one year, after which therapists must renew their certification. Requirements for renewal include abiding by the ARRT ethical standards, paying annual dues, and satisfying continuing education requirements. Continuing education requirements must be met every two years. They require either the completion of 24 course credits related to radiation therapy or the attainment of ARRT certification in a discipline other than radiation therapy. Certification renewal, however, may not be required by all states or by employers that require initial certification.

Licensure

Some states accept ARRT certification as indicating a radiation therapist's qualifications for licensure, but certification doesn't always confer a state license. About two-thirds of the states require radiation therapists to obtain a license from a state accrediting board in addition to certification from ARRT. The license grants radiation therapists permission to work within that state.

For state licensing, ARRT contracts with individual states to administer the exam. Each state has its own rules and procedures for maintaining licensure. This means that radiation therapists may have to pass new state licensure requirements if they move to work in a new state. On occasion, state licensing authorities can arrange for the exam to count for both state licensing and ARRT certification.

Advancement

With additional training and certification, radiation therapists can advance to become medical dosimetrists – technicians who calculate the dose of radiation that will be used for treatment. Other advancement opportunities that may require additional education include teaching, technical sales, and research.

EARNINGS

THE ANNUAL SALARY FOR RADIATION therapists ranges from $50,000 to about $100,000. That works out to be between $24 per hour up to $52 per hour. The median annual wage is about $75,000, or about $36 per hour.

Generally, radiation therapists working for a private practice or company earn more than those employed by public hospitals. Interestingly, radiation therapists employed by smaller clinics earn more on average than those working for larger organizations with more employees. For example, radiation therapists who work for companies with fewer than 200 employees earn a salary of $65,000 to $68,000 per year. Paychecks are slightly bigger – about $70,000 per year – at companies with 600 to 2,000 employees, but at companies with more than 2,000 employees, radiation therapists only earn about $55,000 per year on average.

Salaries vary nationally depending on location, type of facility, industry, and duties. Radiation therapists working in medical and diagnostic laboratories earn the highest salaries on average, while those working in general medical and surgical hospitals typically earn the least. Here are the types of employers and the average annual salaries for radiation therapists working there:

General medical and surgical hospitals: $75,000

Outpatient care centers: $78,000

Offices of physicians: $81,000

Colleges, universities, and professional schools: $84,000

Specialty hospitals (excluding psychiatric and substance abuse facilities): $87,000

Medical and diagnostic laboratories: $91,000

Radiation therapists sometimes go into technical sales. Although the usual reason for making this career change is to earn more money, actual earnings depend upon how much they are able to sell, what commission rates they earn, and the level of demand for their supplies.

As with most professions, salary depends upon job experience. Entry-level radiation therapists who have worked in the field for one year or less have a median salary of about $50,000 per year. Those who have been radiation therapists for one to four years earn about $53,000 per year. Radiation therapists with five to nine years of job experience have salaries of about $65,000 per year. And those with 10 years or more typically make $73,000 to $82,000 per year.

Some employers reimburse their employees for the cost of continuing education. Radiation therapists looking to advance to teaching positions or medical dosimetry may pursue additional job training paid for by their employer.

Annual salaries are also greatly influenced by where radiation therapists work in the country. Radiation therapists working in big cities often earn higher wages than those in less populated locations. For example, the annual mean wage of radiation therapists working in Philadelphia can reach $110,000, and the annual mean wage of radiation therapists in New York City is almost $100,000. However, higher living costs in such metropolitan areas should be taken into account when evaluating the true value of salaries.

Different states vary in how much radiation therapists are paid. Some states may pay less because they have a high concentration of radiation therapists there already, whereas other states may have a greater need of radiation therapists, and will pay more.

Radiation therapists can expect to receive good benefits along with their salary package. Almost all radiation therapists receive healthcare, paid holidays, vacation time, and a retirement plan. Some radiation therapists may receive life insurance or disability, and paid sick leave. Though not as common, radiation therapists may also receive reimbursement for education or training costs, and malpractice insurance.

OPPORTUNITIES

THE JOB OUTLOOK FOR ASPIRING radiation therapists is excellent – far better, in fact, than for most other healthcare professions. Government experts project an increase in the number of radiation therapy positions by almost 30 percent in the coming decade. There are about 15,500 radiation therapists currently employed in the U.S. The National Employment Matrix projects that the number of jobs for radiation therapists will grow to about 20,000 by 2018.

As the population in the United States ages and develops higher risks for cancer, jobs for radiation therapists continue to grow. In addition, as radiation technology becomes safer and more effective, it will be prescribed more often, leading to an increased demand for radiation therapists. In addition to increased demand for radiation therapists, employment growth will result from the need to replace workers who retire or leave the occupation for other reasons.

Job growth is likely to be rapid across all practice settings, including hospitals, physicians' offices, and outpatient centers, but the bulk of job opportunities will continue to be in hospitals. Most radiation therapists – about 70 percent – now work in hospitals, and that is not expected to change in the foreseeable future. The more job openings there are for radiation therapists, the more teaching positions will open up in colleges and universities that offer courses on radiation therapy. The job outlook for medical dosimetry is also good, so radiation therapists who advance to become dosimetrists can expect to find numerous job openings available to them.

Because radiation therapy equipment is very expensive, some hospitals, treatment centers, and insurance companies may try to limit their investments in radiation therapy. This could reduce somewhat the number of radiation therapists needed. Also, if technological advances create programs that perform some of radiation therapist's duties automatically, the demand for these employees could decrease. However, no such technology has yet been developed, and there is no mechanized replacement possible for the therapist-patient interaction that radiation therapists provide.

If an effective treatment plan or cure for cancer other than radiation therapy were to be discovered, there would be less need for radiation therapists. It is difficult to know if or when a better cure for cancer will be found. It is also difficult to determine future cancer rates. As more toxins enter food, water, and air, more and more people may develop cancer, leading to more jobs for radiation therapists.

GETTING STARTED

YOU SHOULD BEGIN ASKING YOURSELF important questions about your future career as a radiation therapist long before you graduate from college or a certificate program. Because radiation therapists must be certified (and in some cases, state licensed) you should consider what state you want to work in so that you can research their requirements. You should also keep track of testing dates for certification and licensure, as these may be offered only a few times per year in your location.

Radiation therapy is a relatively small field. Radiation therapists in the United States hold just over 15,000 jobs. This low number means that you will have to make an effort to seek out radiation therapy communities to network in. Look for any radiation therapy workshops or conferences offered in your area or at your school. The people that you meet there may provide the connections you need to land a job.

Before you attend a workshop or conference, do a little research on the people who are leading it. Then if you get a chance to talk with them directly you will be able to ask detailed questions about their work. Everybody likes to talk about their work – it makes them feel important. More importantly, it shows them how much you care about the field. That deep interest and dedication are important to potential employers.

You should also network with your peers. You may think that it won't help to talk to other prospective radiation therapists, or to radiation therapists who have just entered the field. Those people may not have good connections yet, but someday they may. If they remember you and like you, they might recommend you to someone they know who is in a position to hire you.

It is essential that you stay up to date with the American Registry of Radiologic Technologists (ARRT). The ARRT controls the professional standards required for registration and re-registration of radiation therapists. Anyone working in the field of radiation therapy has gone through testing administered or controlled by the ARRT. This makes it a connecting point for all radiation therapists. The ARRT also provides information and news about the field on its comprehensive website.

The American Society of Radiologic Technologists (ASRT) is another valuable resource. The organization, which describes itself as "The community for radiation technologists," is one that you should join now. The amount of help it can provide in planning and launching your career is amazing. The website provides all sorts of information about upcoming events and conferences, studies and surveys, publications, continuing education, scholarships, and job opportunities. You will even find discounts on hospital dress! Check out the Career Center link on the ASRT website to find current job listings.

There are many ways to track down job opportunities in radiation therapy. You can use employment agencies that specialize in healthcare jobs. You can check the help wanted ads in radiation therapy journals. Your college career counselor can direct you to listings of job openings. Before you apply for any position, make sure your résumé is prepared, that you have letters of recommendation from professors and work supervisors, and that you feel confident speaking about the field and your future role in it.

One of the best ways to prepare for a career in radiation therapy is to find internships that allow you to work in cancer treatment centers alongside real radiation therapists. This will give you an idea of what your days will be like, it will teach you about the field, and it will prepare you for job interviews. When a potential employer asks you specific questions about working as a radiation therapist, you will be able to answer from real life experience rather than what you learned out of a textbook or lecture. You will sound professional, experienced, and ready to begin your career. Plus, your internship might lead to a full-time job after graduation.

ASSOCIATIONS

■ **American Society for Radiation Oncology**
http://www.astro.org

■ **American College of Radiation Oncology**
http://www.acro.org

■ **Association of Freestanding Radiation Oncology Center**
http://www.afroc.org

■ **National Cancer Institute**
http://www.cancer.gov

■ **American Society of Radiologic Technologists**
http://www.asrt.org

■ **American Registry of Radiologic Technologists**
http://www.arrt.org

■ **American Society of Clinical Oncology**
http://www.asco.org

■ **Joint Review Committee on Education in Radiologic Technology**
http://www.jrcert.org

■ **Society of Nuclear Medicine**
http://www.snm.org

PERIODICAL

■ **Radiation Oncology Journal**
http://www.ro-journal.com/content/1/1/2

WEBSITES

■ **Radiation Therapist Jobs**
http://radiationtherapistjobs.org

■ **John Hopkins University**
http://www.radonc.jhmi.edu

■ **The Radiology Student Zone**
http://www.rtstudents.com
/students/index.htm

■ **RadiologyTube.com**
http://www.radiologytube.com

Copyright 2015
Institute For Career Research
Website www.careers-internet.org
For information on other Careers Reports
please contact
service@careers-internet.org

www.ingramcontent.com/pod-product-compliance
Lightning Source LLC
Chambersburg PA
CBHW070744180526
45168CB00004B/1530